STRUGGLING AND WINNING

A Journey Through Death with my Husband

STRUGGLING AND WINNING

A Journey Through Death with my Husband

JANET G. MORRIS

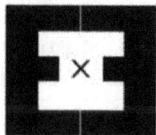

EXPECTED END

ENTERTAINMENT

Atlanta, GA

Published with assistance from Expected End Entertainment
ISBN: 9781737146230

CONTENTS

INTRODUCTION   **1**

Day 1…..3   Day 15…..61   Day 29…..115

Day 2…...7   Day 16…..65   Day 30…..119

Day 3…..11   Day 17…..69   Day 31…..121

Day 4…..15   Day 18….73   Day 32…..125

Day 5…..19   Day 19…..77   Day 33…..133

Day 6…..23   Day 20…..81   Day 34…..137

Day 7…..27   Day21…..85   Day 35…..141

Day 8…..31   Day 22….89   Day 36…..145

Day 9…..37   Day 23…..93   Day 37…..149

Day 10….41   Day 24…..97   Day 38…..153

Day 11….45   Day 25…..101   Day 39…..157

Day 12….49   Day 26…..105   Day 40…..161

Day 13….53   Day 27….109   Day 41…..165

Day 14….57   Day 28…..111

DEDICATION

This book is dedicated to my late husband Tyree Morris, Jr. His love for me and his determination to see Jesus brought more intimacy to our marriage and caused a transformation in me that I never could have imagined.

INTRODUCTION

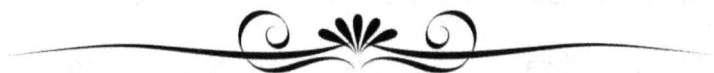

To write this book, I had to dig deep into my soul, my spiritual being, and talk only to God.

I listened to my sisters, Betty and Susan, who told me for years, "You should write a book. There is a book in you. You should put this in a book."

To my granddaughter, Genesis Marie, who said, "This belongs in a book Gran, a two-part book."

So, here we go with the guidance of the Holy Spirit and a talk with my Pastor Jon Shorterez, whom I trust to direct me spiritually on the new journey of pouring out and sharing the goodness of God. What do I have to lose?

Okay God, I hear you. So, here I go... I am in your powerful hands.

DAY ONE

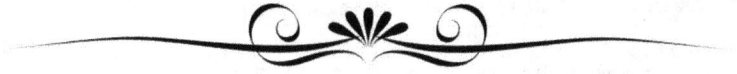

Day 1

Life-Changing Circumstances

Entreat me not to leave you... Ruth 1:16

Hi, my name is Janet M. I am a widow. My husband died of dementia on March 12, 2012, and six months later, I was diagnosed with Congestive Heart Failure (CHF) and Arterial Fibrillation. I had to get an electrical shock to get my heart back on a proper beat. WOW!!!

As the years rolled by, I was diagnosed with other diseases such as diabetes, high blood pressure, kidney failure, anemia, high cholesterol, lesions on my liver, low blood pressure, possible cancer, possible lupus, parathyroid issues, neuropathy, arthritis, and finally edema in my legs, stomach, hands, and fingers. With all these things going on, I am still winning. How?

Being too active causes edema leading to an increase of fluid in my body, resulting in swelling in the legs, stomach, hands, and fingers... sometimes with pain. When this occurs, I must slow down, rest and stay close to the bed so the fluid can release quickly... with the help of medicine. However, I am still winning.

I am constantly changing my eating habits. My taste buds continue to change daily. I exercise when possible; disappointed when I can't. I miss out on family outings and/or celebrations. If I attend or participate in any of these activities, I run the risk of fluid buildup that can affect my heart and cause me to be hospitalized. This is a daily struggle of choosing the right food and choosing what activity I can do each day that will not cause fluid retention or cause my heart to beat at a rapid pace.

My life is not the same as it was nine years and seven months ago, not even 22 years ago. This year, my husband and I would have been married for 22 years this past June 10. He was diagnosed with early dementia in 2007 and progressively got worse the next year. That's when my wedding vows to him got serious. It stuck in my mind and would not leave. ("For better or worse, for richer or poorer; in sickness and in health; to death us do part.") Struggling and Winning.

Short Prayer

Dear God, master of the universe, I need you to help me make it through all of this. I am not strong without you. Your words say when I am weak your strength is made perfect in me. I trust that you will give me the strength to endure.

Scripture

And He said to me, "My grace is sufficient for you, for My strength is made perfect in weakness… (NKJV)

2 Corinthians 12: 9

DAY TWO

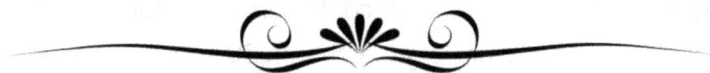

Day 2

Committed to the Vow

"May the God of hope fill you with all joy and peace in believing, so that by power of the Holy Spirit you may abound in Hope." (Romans 15:13 ESV)

The marriage vows I took with my husband and in front of over 100 witnesses on June 10, 2000, pushed me to focus on the only one I knew who could carry us through this struggle, who was none other than JESUS, my Lord and Savior. Those words (the vows) resonated in my Spirit with every deed, action, and step I made to make my husband's life on earth as comfortable as possible. And so did Psalm 23 (The Lord is my Shepherd) and Psalm 27 (The Lord is my light and my Salvation).

I heard stories about people with dementia not remembering their loved ones, changes in attitude, the caregiver struggling with the patient to get them to do what is best for them. Everything they normally do for themselves becomes a challenge, from feeding themselves, bathing themselves, dressing themselves, and grooming themselves. Those responsibilities fall to the caregiver. It is like having a newborn baby. It reminds me of the old Proverb that says, "Once a man, twice a child." The theory of retro-genesis is simple.

Love kept us together. Love strengthened me through this struggle causing me to win each step each day. Did it look like I was winning? Maybe not to others, and sometimes not even to me. But, as I reflect on the things that transpired during those four years of Tyree's depleting health, God was there all the time. He was holding us together and making our love stronger. He helped me to fulfill the promise I made to Tyree, which was to love him unconditionally no matter what, and to remember Corinthians 13. I realized that it wasn't me; it was God in me. What do I mean?

God is part of us because we are made in his image (Genesis 1:26-28; Genesis 2:7). He breathed the breath of life in us, and we became living souls. The Spirit of the living God is on the inside of me that helps me to do His will when I yield to him and follow his command.

Short Prayer

Father God, I need you to help me to keep the vow I made to Tyree. Help me to show your love toward him no matter the circumstances. Help me to stand like the wife I ask you to help me to be. God, you said, "I will never leave you nor forsake you." I need you right now.

Scripture

"...Be strong and courageous and do the work. Do not be afraid or discouraged, for the Lord God, my God is with you. He will not fail you nor forsake you until all the work for the service of the temple of the Lord is finished." 1 Chronicles 28:20 ESV

DAY THREE

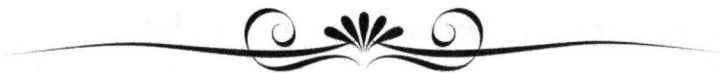

Day 3

Another Chance

"When the Spirit of Truth comes, he will guide you into all the truth, ... and he will declare to you the things that are to come." (John16:13 ESV)

Believe me when I say, it was all God. I had been here before – married – but did not do the "for better or worse". I did not want to, and I did not ask God to help me do the "worse" part (I had no idea what worse was). God gave me another chance to show that I could do what he created me to do. All I had to do was lean on him, not the world, not family and friends' ideas or suggestions. I needed God's strength to make it through this journey.

This journey was not expected, it was not something I thought I was prepared for, but it was a path that God knew Tyree and I was going to take long before we were born. God knew our response to the doctor's diagnosis. He knew how Tyree and I would handle the diagnosis of early signs of dementia. He knew Tyree would not want to live dependent on others for his basic needs. He knew I had the strength to go through it all. I had no clue.

It reminds me of Jeremiah when God told him, "I knew you before you were formed in your mother's womb". Also, "I know the plans and thoughts I have for you". (Jeremiah 1:5 and Jeremiah 29:11) Throughout the diagnosis, the deteriorating, the drama, and the ups and downs of this disease, God knew everything. He knew how to hold us together with His love. He reminded us how much we loved each other, how strong our love was, and the promises we made to each other.

Tyree and I got closer on the path that led to death for both of us. Tyree experienced a physical death and I experienced a spiritual death. He was being prepared for transition. I was preparing to be born again. Jesus talks about being born again with Nicodemus. John 3:3 says, "Except man/woman be born again he/she cannot see the kingdom of God." We both wanted to see the kingdom of God. I wanted to get this path of marriage correct this time. I did not ask God if I could leave. Instead, I accepted the word that God gave me in August 2011.

With the medical diagnosis hanging over our heads, we did not want to accept it, especially Tyree. He did not like it when I had to ask for his car keys or me telling the doctors how his week went. Tyree most definitely did not like it when the caregiver came to assist him with his daily hygiene even though he was a man. It got hard for me to help him because he was dead weight. The doctor told me I needed to get some assistance because he was unable to walk or get up out of the bed to sit in his wheelchair.

He went from a man filled with energy to a man with the mind of an infant who had no clue on how to do anything for himself. It's the life Tyree did not want. For me to see him deteriorate like that was hard and unbelievable. I could not imagine what was going through his mind the times he would pick up the fork to feed himself and then put the fork back down. He'd stare as if to say, "Why can't I feed myself? I want to, but my cognitive skills are not cooperating."

This was the man I grew to love. I loved laugh, his voice, his protection, and his expressions of love. But he was no longer able to do these things. God, how do I handle this and what do I say to family members? Some of them didn't believe the things I told them about Tyree, that he was not getting any better.

How do I communicate medical updates without causing drama?

God said, "Just remember what I told you and do it."

But God, you already know who is going to have an issue with the medical report that I am about to give.

God said, "I can handle it and so can you. I am right here with you."

Short Prayer

Father God, creator of heaven and earth, I need you to take control of my tongue so I can say what you say. I need my flesh to take a seat and the Holy Ghost to rise up in me and speak in Jesus' name.

Scripture

"I said, I will guard my ways that I may not sin with my tongue…" (Psalm 39:1 ESV)

DAY FOUR

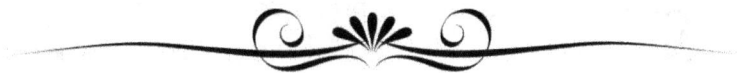

Day 4

Trusting God's Voice

"Son of man, behold, I am about to take the delight of your eyes away...yet you shall not mourn or weep, nor shall your tears run down." (Ezekiel 24:16 ESV)

Everyone is not going to agree with how I followed the instructions of God. But that is okay. God rewarded me for following His instructions. He prepared me for my husband's death. God told me that this sickness would overtake my husband and that he was going to die.

When I initially heard God talking to me, I did not take it seriously. That is until God told me a third time. He said, "Janet." Immediately, I got up and wrote down everything He said. He spoke of how everything would transpire; when to tell others; what my husband would wear when he died; what I would wear to the funeral; the color of the casket; and how the funeral service would be. God said, *"You will not mourn like others. It will seem strange to some. They will think that you are not grieving."* As God was telling me this, I thought about what He told Ezekiel in the bible when his wife died: *"Son of man, behold, I am about to take the delight of your eyes away...yet you shall not mourn or weep, nor shall your tears run down."*

What about going through the death journey? What is worse? What was worse?

According to dictionary.com:

Worse: adjective of poorer quality or lower standard; less good or desirable; more ill or unhappy.

Verb: less well or skillfully

The definition of worse describes what Tyree experienced prior to his death. The quality of his life was poor. There was no more mowing the lawn, washing the car, cleaning the house, kissing, cuddling, tight hugs, cooking dinners together, and making decisions. There was no more saying I love you, singing or whistling. There was no more walking cool when he wore a suit, no more surprises lying on the bed after I had worked all day, and no more greeting me at the door with hugs and kisses. NO MORE!!!

All of these moments had vanished, but I had to keep moving forward knowing one day Tyree was going to leave me here on this earth. I did not know the exact day, but I knew it was getting closer. I was unable to tell everyone about the four conversations God had with me. I had to go on like a loving wife. The hardest part was not being able to share this with anyone. I had no issue with loving Tyree completely. However, I was surprised that I wasn't trying to figure out a way to leave him in his condition. I was totally committed to being a loving wife all way through the process because this was Tyree's choice and God shared His thoughts with me.

Short Prayer

Dear Heavenly Father, this is hard for me. I realize that I

have to follow your instructions, but this thing is hard, and I want to do your will, nevertheless. I know you do all things great. So, please help me to hold to your promise of peace, even if the peace does not look the way I think it should. In Jesus' name.

Scripture

"Saying, Father, if thou be willing, remove this cup from me: nevertheless, not my will, but thine, be done." (Luke 22:42 KJV)

DAY FIVE

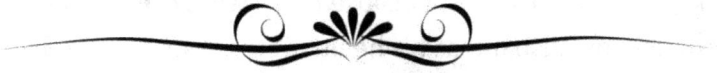

Day 5

Staying Connected

"Abide in me, and I in you. As the branch cannot bear fruit by itself, unless it abides in the vine, neither can you, unless you abide in me." (John 15:4ESV)

What am I supposed to do as his health declines? I still believed that God would be with me every step of the way. Was it hard? Yes, because there were others who did not see my husband as his health deteriorated. They did not believe the medical reports I was giving them. I always turn to the Lord for strength to keep going. I relied on Jesus to lead me all the way. I prayed a lot. I called on Jesus a lot. Sometimes, I would only say, "Jesus, Jesus, Jesus, I cannot do this unless you help me." When I said this, I would remember his words, *"I will never leave you nor forsake you."* (Matthew 28:20b; Deuteronomy 31:8)

Short Prayer

Father God, I need your help to remain connected to you. This is extremely hard. I am seeking you according to Matthew 6:33: *"Seek ye, first the kingdom of God and his righteousness…"* Please, help me to stay connected to you. In Jesus' name, Amen.

Scripture

"Abide in me, and I in you. As the branch cannot bear fruit

by itself, unless it abides in the vine, neither can you, unless you abide in me." (John 15:4 ESV)

JANET G. MORRIS

DAY SIX

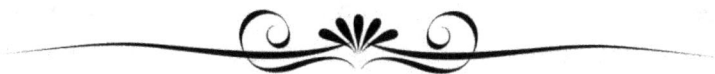

Day 6

Pressing My Way Through

"The spirit indeed is willing, but the flesh is weak".
Matthew 26:41(ESV)

Tyree's disease prepared me for my sickness. It taught me how to be obedient and disciplined, to be committed and willing. It taught me how to press my way through after hearing each doctor's report. It pushed me to rely on God every time and every day. It built me up to trust God more and more by showing me just how much I needed God to go through it all, no matter how painful/hurtful. Issues with doctors and nurses helped me to recognize who God really is. During the process, I learned more about Him and just how much He cared for Tyree and cares for me; how much he loved Tyree and loves me; and how much he was looking out for Tyree and me.

God's love was shown through this course, and He was there all the time. I could not allow outside interference to cause me to stray away from God. To help Tyree, I had to yell for Jesus' name many times. Some days, I would forget to say, "Come, Jesus, come with me. If you do not come with me, I am going to mess up." I would go back to the starting point and ask Jesus to come with me. I invited Jesus in every time. Yes, it was hard, but I did anyway. If it wasn't for Jesus, I would not have been able to withstand so many negative things that were being said to me or behind my back.

As the artist Andrae Crouch sang, "Through it all, I have learned to depend upon His Word." It was God almighty leading and guiding me all the way. God is AWESOME!!!

Short Prayer

Father God, you are holy and there is no one like you. No one can take your place. Thank you for always being there helping through my weakness every second, minute, hour, and day.

Scripture

"When I am weak His strength is made perfect in me." (2 Corinthians 12:9)

JANET G. MORRIS

DAY SEVEN

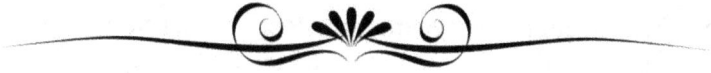

Day 7

Just to Be in His Presence

"...and the peace of God will guard your heart and minds in Christ Jesus." (Philippians 4:7 ESV)

I've had the opportunity to feel His presence so strongly, to feel Him carrying me, holding me up, hugging me, and holding my hands. He allowed me to lay my head on His shoulders and in His lap. Tyree's death and my sickness has caused me to have a closer walk with Jesus. My faith has increased. My wisdom, knowledge, and understanding have increased. My ears are opened to His voice. My soul yearns more and more each day to be in the presence of God.

When you hear ministers, pastors, or worshippers speak about being in the presence of God and how it makes them do things that you do not understand, it is because you have never experienced it. You cannot imagine that such a thing can happen. Well, let me tell you I am a witness. Being in the presence of God is not understandable if you're not in the Spirit. *"The natural person does not accept the things of the Spirit of God, for they are folly to him, and he is not able to understand them because they are spiritually discerned."* (I Corinthians 2:14 ESV).

Another scripture to support that the carnal minded person cannot understand the Spirit of God is, Romans 8

(KJV) Because the carnal mind is an enmity against God; for it is not subject to the law of God, neither indeed can be. Therefore, my ability is not what gets me in the presence of God, it is the Holy Spirit that leads me to the presence of God. I must accept the Spirit of God that leads me toward the will of God. God promises that he will keep me in perfect peace if I keep my mind stayed on him and the peace of God will guard your heart and minds in Christ Jesus *(Isaiah 26:3; Philippians 4:7ESV)*

If my mind stays on Jesus, I trust him to keep me no matter what I am going through, dealing with or confronting. Jesus' peace is with me because I trust His will, His thoughts, and His plans for me. I trust Him because my faith is in Him (God).

Short Prayer

Lord, thank you, for helping me to remain in your presence so I can keep my eyes stayed on you. Thank you, for keeping me in perfect peace. Thank you for keeping your word and it not returning void. Being in your presence is where I feel the calmest.

Scripture

"You keep in perfect peace those whose mind is stayed on you because he trusts in you." (Isaiah 26:3 ESV)

DAY EIGHT

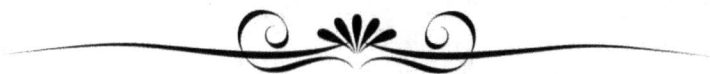

Day 8

Letting Go

"Cast your burden on the Lord, and he will sustain you..."
(Psalm 55:22 ESV)

I had to let go of my feelings and ask God to guide me through everything. I had to constantly give my burdens to the Lord. I could not handle things by myself or of my own strength.

- Tyree's sickness/disease
- Taking care of him
- Talking to doctors
- Keeping him at home or letting him go to the hospital or nursing home
- Talking to family members, friends, apostles, pastors
- Making sure he was taken care of properly by the medical providers
- Saying no when I wanted to say yes.
- Keeping Tyree's wishes (it was most definitely a struggle)

None of these were easy, but with God it was peaceful and joyful. It was peaceful because I was equipped to fulfill the wishes of my husband even though they were not *my* wishes. Tyree was ready to go to be with Jesus. He was very sure about it once his dementia got worse. It was all he could think about, "I want to see Jesus." He told me of the things he saw: a field full of flowers and butterflies flying around and Jesus at the foot of his hospital bed. He said, "I miss my mama and my daddy."

Every day as God promised, he was there for me and Tyree. He made it so peaceful. I leaned on God and trusted that he knew what was best for Tyree and me. He wanted both of us to be at peace. I followed His instructions as hard as it was. There was still peace for Tyree and me. He honored Tyree's wish and not mine. I had to accept Tyree's wish to die. God promised to keep me in perfect peace if I kept my mind stayed on him.

I wanted Tyree to live a long life but that was not my decision to make. It was not my body that the illness was taking over; the body that was deteriorating was Tyree's. Therefore, it was his decision to choose how he wanted to live the rest of his days on earth. Before he could no longer think for himself, we discussed death. He was ready to die; and I was not ready for that. Even though God warned me of Tyree's death approximately 6 months prior to Tyree's death. I had to accept it with the help of God.

When God initially told me about the death of Tyree, I could not tell anyone. God released me to tell others (certain people) in stages about the conversations I had with Him. Prior to God telling me about Tyree's death, we had to tell his children about the dementia. It was on Thanksgiving the year before he died. Because Tyree did not want to tell them, it was a struggle to determine when to do so. The reason I wanted them to inform them was so they wouldn't be upset with for not knowing. God helped with this as well.

This journey was a struggle, but I am winning all the way. God was with me every single day I allowed Him in to help me grieve, according to His plan. Going through Tyree's sickness prepared me for my illness and inability to do the things I was able to do before. The fact that I still have my being is a plus. I may not be able to do things the way I used to, be as active as I once was, or maintain a job, but God is looking after me. I have not wanted for anything.

I am winning despite the struggles. God is holding me up because of a decision to allow Him to be the head of my life. I take no credit for anything. I give God all the glory and honor for showing his love towards me and Tyree. Tyree is not suffering anymore; he is in a safe place waiting for Jesus to return for his church. I am on earth striving to live daily in the will of the Lord.

Short Prayer

Father God, I really need you to keep me and help me to deal with all these issues. Without you my flesh is going to rise causing me to be out of your will. I need to feel your presence and hear your voice filled with directions and words to respond to all people as well as make the right decision on Tyree's behalf. I ask that you do not leave nor forsake me.

Scripture

"Sustain me, my God, according to your promise, and I will

live, do not let my hopes be dashed." (Psalm 119:116 NLTV)

JANET G. MORRIS

DAY NINE

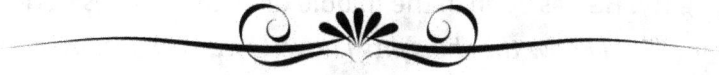

Day 9

He is a Keeper

"The Lord watches over you-the Lord is your shade at your right hand…" **(Psalm 121: 5 NIV)**

God is keeping me. He keeps on holding me up, daily. He is being God all through my struggles, my pain, my heartaches, my ups, and my downs. God is showing he is mighty. He has been in the middle of all things considering me. *"For I know the thoughts I have toward you, saith the Lord, thoughts of peace, and not of evil, to give you and expected end." (Jeremiah 29:11 KJV)*

Struggling with God beside you is better than struggling alone. The pain and hurt are there along with disappointments, confusion, and misunderstanding. But God will help us if we lean on Him and if we call upon His name. He is always ready to intercede on our behalf. We must believe that, walk in faith, and trust in His word.

Tyree's death was also my death journey. Why? Because, I had to watch a piece of my husband die each day until he was gone. I had to see a healthy, intelligent, confident young man forget how to take care of himself. He was a proud man being reduced to a baby mentality, a baby with no sense of direction or understanding the need to bathe, brush his teeth, go to the restroom, or feed himself.

We were being transformed into how God saw us, not how we saw each other. What God saw was better than what we saw. God saw us suffering together as husband and wife. God saw in us a love that was unconditional. We were made for such a time as this. Who knew? God did. He knew the pain that would come with death. Tyree was dying physically, and I was dying spiritually. It was painful letting things happen according to God's will and Tyree's wishes.

Short Prayer

Father God, thank you for helping me to follow your instructions. Thank you, for your comfort, peace, and joy. Your joy is what gives me strength to keep moving toward you for further instructions. Your plans are perfect.

Scripture

"...Do not be grieved, for the joy of the LORD is your strength. (Nehemiah 8:10b NIV)

DAY TEN

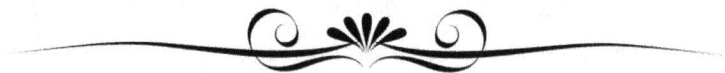

Day 10

Producing while Going Through

"But the fruit of the Spirit is love, joy, peace, forbearance, kindness, goodness, faithfulness, gentleness and self-control. Against such things there is no law."
Gal. 5:22-23 (NIV)

Tyree and I began one when we said our vows. We became one according to the word of God. Tyree's death caused me to die to selfishness. His death made be more patient, understanding, and compassionate. I was able to do so with the assistance of the Holy Spirit to produce the fruit of the Spirit that the Bible speaks about in Galatians 5:22-24.

The fruit of the Spirit is:

- Love
- Joy
- Peace
- Patience
- Kindness
- Goodness
- Faithfulness
- Gentleness
- Self-control

Against such there is no law. Those who belong to Christ Jesus have crucified the flesh with its passions and desires.

I had to let my passions and desires die. I could no longer hold on to what I wanted for Tyree, for him to continue to live and not die right now. I had promised Tyree I would do what he desired. Was it hard? Yes. Was it a struggle? Yes. Was it more than I thought I could bear? Yes. But because of Jesus leading me every step of the way, it was also easy. Why was it easy? As the years passed, I realized the Holy Spirit handled the hard part, leading me to the word of God. My flesh wanted to say forget all this, but my Spirit would not allow me to do it. You can handle this, really??? I surrendered to the will of God.

Short Prayer

Thank you, God for comforting me through my tribulation. Giving me the strength to move forward when my flesh did not want to and the Spirit on the inside of me did.

Scripture

"Who comforted us in all tribulation, that we may be able to comfort them which are in any trouble, by the comfort wherewith we ourselves are comforted of God." (2 Corinthians 1:4 ESV)

DAY ELEVEN

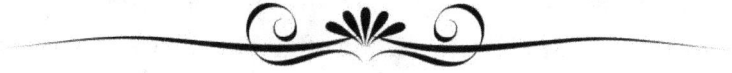

Day 11

Realty Check

"Watch and pray, that ye enter not into temptation; the Spirit indeed is willing, but the flesh is weak."
(Matthew 26:41 KJV)

As each day passed, I would think about the goodness of Jesus and how He was by my side every step of the way as He promised. This strengthened my love for Tyree, the love I had committed to in June of 2000. I realize that it was God's grace and mercy that kept me going daily. The mercy of God is new every day. *"The steadfast love of the Lord never ceases: his mercies never come to an end: they are new every morning: great is His faithfulness."* (Lamentations 3: 22- 23 ESV)

I understand that I am still here because of the grace of God. God loves me. God is concerned about me, the whole me. God shows Himself to me every day, all day. For me to see God orchestrating this event, I had to be connected to His Spirit. I had to yield myself to His Spirit. I have heard it said, "Man cannot dwell in the Spirit for too long." I do not understand the meaning of that statement. The Bible says it is the Spirit that leads us into all truth and to walk in the Spirit and do not fulfill the lust of the flesh; do not quench the Holy Spirit. (John 16:13; Galatians 5:16; 1 Thessalonians 5:19) Therefore, we need the Holy Spirit to guide us so we can do what the word of God says to do.

I would not have been able to care for and love my sweet-cakes the way I did; it was all God. It was His strength, His joy and His words that led me in the right direction. Did my flesh, my own thoughts want to take over? Absolutely, but it was not about me; it was about Tyree. I needed the Holy Spirit to lead me in taking care of Tyree with love and compassion while allowing God's and Tyree's will to be followed and not my own.

Every day, my will weakened, dying so God's will could direct me.   The Spirit is always ready to do as the will of God suggests, but the flesh is weak when it comes to doing the will of the Lord.

Short Prayer

Father God, thank you! I can always count on you to help me to follow you. I accept that my flesh is weak, but my Spirit is ready to follow your instructions. Thank you for placing your Spirit inside of me to help me follow your prefect will.

Scripture

"Howbeit when he, the Spirit of truth is come, he will guide you into all truth..." (John 16:13 KJV)

JANET G. MORRIS

DAY TWELVE

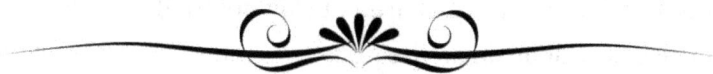

Day 12

Dealing with Death

"Blessed are they that mourn, for they shall be comforted."
(Matthew 5:4 KJV)

Yes, it is hard to see a loved one die. I watched my stepfather die, which was very emotional and draining. It was a rollercoaster experience. I did not know the body could endure what transpired during death. It was also a release and cleansing... the hollering, the shaking of the body, the tears and the snot running down your face. After releasing my emotions, my body felt relaxed, light, and I was sad.

Tyree's death was totally different for me because God prepared me for his death. I would not have received this *special* message from God about Tyree's death if I were not connected to Him, His Spirit. I did not cry uncontrollably, which was a surprise to me. I shouted at his funeral because I was overjoyed about how God had orchestrated everything from when to tell people about Tyree's health, when to give updates, what clothes to prepare for Tyree's funeral, what I was going to wear, the color of the casket, the songs that would be sung, the time the funeral was to be held... everything! It was like going wherever the wind blew, like a leaf on the street pushed by the wind.

Short Prayer

Thank you God for showing your love toward me and Tyree. You stood right there and helped in every way. You held my hand while guiding my heart and mind. You aided me through something I consider worse. Father God, you made me stand in awe of you. I thank you, from the bottom of my heart to the depth of my soul.

Scripture

"Blessed are they that mourn they shall be comforted." (Matthew 5:4 KJV)

JANET G. MORRIS

DAY THIRTEEN

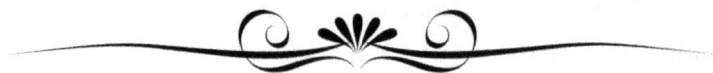

Day 13

A God Connection

"Trust in the Lord with all thine heart…" (Proverbs 3:5 NIV)

The wind in my life is the Holy Spirit. It is the wind of God directing me all the way. I was winning because I was following the will of God on this death journey. It caused God to do just what he said he would do. *"Trust in the Lord with all your heart, and do not lean on your own understanding. In all your ways acknowledge him, and he will make straight your paths. Be not wise in your own eyes; fear the Lord and turn away from evil. It will be health to your flesh and refreshment to your bones."* (Proverbs 3:5-8 ESV) I trusted God to do just what he said he would do.

It is still amazing to me that God would tell me that he would prepare me for everything I was going to face concerning Tyree. This is what God means when he said, "Lo I am with you always, even unto the end of the earth…" (Matthew 28:20b)

God's steadfast love for me guided me every step of the way. God helped me endure things I never thought I could. He helped me stand in the fire and come out as pure gold. He continues to show himself in my life. God is more than I could ever imagine. My mind cannot comprehend the total greatness of God. Every time He shows himself, it is greater than the time before. No one can outdo God, the father of Abraham, Isaac, and Jacob... the Creator of the Heavens and the Earth.

Short Prayer

Father God, you are so amazing. Oh, how I trust you to take good care of me. Oh, how I trust your thoughts and plans for me. I trust that you will do just what you said. I appreciate your steadfast love.

Scripture

"For I know the plans I have for you, declares the Lord..." (Jeremiah 29:11 NIV)

JANET G. MORRIS

DAY FOURTEEN

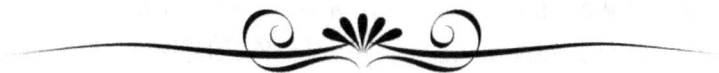

Day 14

The Pain of Death

"O death, where is your victory? O death, where is your sting?" (I Corinthians 15:55 ESV)

The more I look back and think about Tyree's sickness and how God stayed with him and I through it all, the more I am thankful for God. He helped Tyree deal with the pain of death. It was so *INCREDIBLE*. Tyree never asked for pain medication. The hospice nurse said that the pain associated with death sometimes causes patients to cry out for the strongest medicines, like morphine, but Tyree never did. He lay in his bed yielding to everything so his soul could be released to Jesus. Tyree never complained; his death was peaceful, just the way he wanted. Tyree knew I could handle his death more than he could handle mine. I used to think he was crazy, but not anymore.

Even though I had Tyree's wishes in writing, I still had to take a stand and express his concerns, wants, and desires to every medical provider. I would ask each time, "Don't you have the medical directive in his chart? I should not have to repeat myself every time I come into this establishment." Yet I did… every time. This was more draining than taking care of Tyree at home.

Through it all, I learned to depend on God. Some days I would just say, "Jesus, Jesus, Jesus! I cannot do this without your help." I would then go on and follow the directions of the Holy Spirit.

As you read this book you may have many questions as to why things happened the way they did. I don't have answers for you. God works in mysterious ways to perform wonders. I have learned that according to the word of God (which I strive to follow daily), God's thoughts are not our thoughts; His ways are not our ways. His thoughts are higher than mine and ours. (Romans 11: 33-36; Isaiah 55:8-9)

You see, I have committed myself to be a servant of the Lord. The inheritance I have is that God's gotten me through everything... trials, temptations, criticism, the mean looks, all the murmuring and complaining based on Tyree's wishes. God walked with me through it all. If He didn't, I would have been "like a ship without a sail".

Short Prayer

Father God, I am so grateful to you that you stayed with me. Even though there were times that I thought I could not make it, you reminded me of the promise you made that you would be right there. God, you are truly an awesome God. No one can take your place.

Scripture

"But thanks be to God! He gives us the victory through our Lord Jesus Christ." (I Corinthians 15:57 NIV)

DAY FIFTEEN

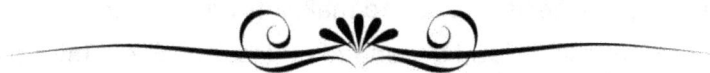

Day 15

Committing to the Lord with my Mouth and Action

"Commit thy way unto the Lord; trust also in him; and he shall bring it to pass." (Psalm 37:5 KJV)

Committing to the Lord was and is the best thing that has ever happened to me. Knowing that God was there leading and guiding me all the way helped me to be at peace about every decision I had to make on Tyree's behalf. I called on Jesus a lot. I depended on Jesus to direct my path on this death journey. "Yea though I walk through the valley of the shadow of death, I will fear no evil: for thou are with me; thy rod and thy staff they comfort me..." (Psalm 23:4 KJV)

When God first told me Tyree was going to die, His voice was so soft, sweet, and gentle. *"Janet, Tyree is going to get worse and die."* God had to tell me three times before I came to the realization that it was truly God speaking. The death journey began along with the ups and downs, crying, craziness, unbelievable attitudes, stress, frustration, misunderstandings, and so much stress. I was only able to handle the drama with the help of the Lord.

God is AWESOME!!! The words on these pages cannot express the goodness of the Lord and all that He has done and continue to do for me. I am searching for words to give you a clear, detailed description of how God showed up in my life during this death journey with my Sweet-cakes. I am not able to find words in the English dictionary. What I can say is that it was so **amazing**! It was more than amazing how God orchestrated everything.

Short Prayer

Father God, you're so amazing. You're awesome. Words cannot express how grateful I am for your love toward me and Tyree. You have not left us alone. You're allowing Tyree to die in peace and helping me to be at peace. What a mighty God you are.

Scripture

"The Lord is my rock, and my fortress, any my deliverer; my God, my strength, in whom I will trust; my buckler, and the horn of my salvation, and my high tower." (Psalm 18:2 KJV)

DAY SIXTEEN

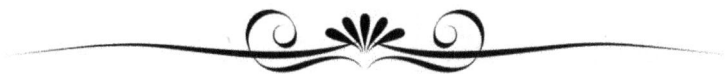

Day 16

Amazing???

"Even though I walk through the valley of the shadow of death, I will fear no evil, for thy are with me thy rod and staff, they comfort me." (Psalm 23:4 ESV)

I did not think it was amazing while going through Tyree's death. I was calling on the Lord along with reaching out to prayer warriors, intercessors, apostles, and prophets to pray for me, encourage me, and give me spiritual advice. These people led me back to God.

The pain of grief is no joke. It comes when you least expect it. It shows up like an unexplainable pain in your body. Pain comes in many forms, like when you are walking down the street and you see or smell something that reminds you of the individual who has died. Or, when you are cooking dinner and you remember the time you prepared that meal together. Or, when are looking at a television show you enjoyed together. The pain of grief causes you to slow down your daily activities when these thoughts come. You try everything you can to push through the pain. It is very frustrating trying to explain the pain and emotions surrounding what you're feeling. You try to talk about it, read scriptures, pray, meditate, and cry. Many things occur without a clear way to explain those feelings to others, especially when the person is not really listening or can't relate to what you are going through.

I can now see the hands of God was in it all. It was evident in how he carried me, taught me, helped me, held me up, wrapped me in his loving arms and never left my side. He helped me to keep my mind stayed on him. God backed up His word: *"I will keep you in perfect peace if you keep your mind stayed on me."* I trusted him to lead and guide me all the way. *"Thou will keep him in perfect peace, whose mind is stayed on thee; because he trusteth in thee."* (Isaiah 26:3 KJV)

I am at peace after my death journey; and it is all thanks to God. I still have some days where I ask myself, "Are you really at peace with everything that occurred during Tyree's sickness and death?" I give God all credit for my peace because I continue to keep my mind stayed on Him.

Short Prayer

Lord, I praise you and honor you for keeping me in perfect peace as I keep my mind stayed on you. You are most certainly the Great I AM. You are everything I need to continue this journey. Thank you, God, for your rod and staff that comfort me.

Scripture

"...for thou art with me; thy rod and thy staff comfort me." (Psalm 23:4 KJV)

DAY SEVENTEEN

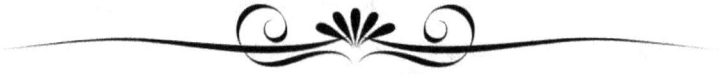

Day 17

Tyree's Decision

"Have not I commanded you? Be strong, vigorous, and very courageous. Be not afraid, neither be dismayed, for the Lord your God is with you wherever you go."
(Joshua 1:9 AMP)

Tyree was struggling more than I was. I could imagine him thinking, "Is Janet going to honor my wishes? How can I live just a little bit longer for those who are not ready for me to leave?" I saw him struggling to remain alive and struggling to die because that is what he really desired. After speaking with the hospice nurse, she confirmed what the Holy Spirit was telling me.

I learned that the fleshly body is in pain when death is near. The more the body tries to hold on to life, the more severe the pain. Releasing the person to move on to death eases that pain. I gave Tyree my word that I would do everything I could to honor his wishes. I told him that I was okay and would be okay. Did it hurt to say those words to him? It most certainly did! I did not keep my word immediately, but with the help of God, I did... eventually. It took approximately two months for me to completely get in line with God. It took a lot of praying. After I told Tyree I was with his desire to die, his body immediately began to relax. I could see a smile on his face. It looked like his skin was glowing.

Many questions raced through my mind: How can this be? What is going on? How can I go on without a clear explanation?

The decline in Tyree's intellect and cognitive functions happened so fast. At the same time, the days seemed to drag by. The process took seven months from August 2011 to March 2012. With each doctor visit, hospital stay, and nursing homes, he was deteriorating from the man I married to an infant. He went from being independent to not knowing what being independent was; from talking to not talking; to not opening his eyes; to not wanting to move any parts of his body; to not sitting up or standing up or walking.

Short Prayer

Dear God, this is so devastating. Tyree does not want to do anything but lie in bed. I no longer have the strength to take care of him alone at home. I do not want him to go to a nursing home. Whatever your will is I am willing to do it with your help. I need your help to make this decision and your strength to accept/embrace the decision, in Jesus' name.

Scripture

"...My Father if it be possible, let this cup pass from me; nevertheless, not as I will, but as you will." (Matthew 26:39 ESV)

JANET G. MORRIS

DAY EIGHTEEN

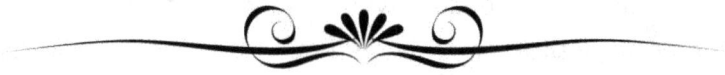

Day 18

Tyree's Struggle

"We are confident, I say, and willing rather to be absent from the body, and to be present with the Lord." (2 Corinthians 5:8 (KJV)

I really did not realize how much Tyree was struggling until I put pen to paper for this book. I was not the only one struggling. He was dealing with the doctors, nurses, therapists, visitors (friends and family members), as well as me. He was also going through the pain of going back and forth to home, hospital, nursing home, hospital, home, hospital, nursing home, etc.

Since he was not able to dress himself or clean himself, it took a lot out of him. He took pride in how he looked. The swag when he walked was not there anymore. His smile and voice had faded away. He no longer whistled at me or like he did while he worked. He stopped singing. The joy of living was no longer present. It all disappeared like day turning to night, the sun going down and darkness appearing.

What I love about him is that he was brave through it all. He was humble. He never complained or murmured about being in pain. He had the opportunity to request morphine, but never did. He was struggling to get to the place he desired to go because there were people who were not ready for him to die.

I promised to take him as my husband. I pledged my life and love to him in the name of the Father, the Son, and the Holy Spirit. I made a commitment to my Sweet-cakes, whom I knew to be level-headed, sharp, smart, intelligent, clever, witty, and charming. He used to be a fixer, but after getting sick, he couldn't even figure out how to hold a spoon or fork to feed himself. This is what God meant when he said, "Tyree sickness will get worse and then he will die, but his death will be peaceful." WOW!

My Sweet-cakes was fading away in front of my very eyes and there was nothing I could do about it. All I could do was honor the vows we said to each other in June 2000. I promised to love, honor, trust, and to be with him in sickness and in health, in adversity, in prosperity, to cleave only to him until death parted us.

We both recited Ruth 1:16 (ESV):

"But Ruth said, 'Do not urge me to leave you or to return from following you. Fore where you go I will go, and where you lodge I will lodge. Your people shall be my people, and your God my God.'"

Short Payer

Thank you, Lord, for allowing me this opportunity to love and cherish Tyree. You made this love extra special for us. Father God, you helped us to get through the rough times of our marriage, together. You allowed us another chance to stay committed to our vows. We made those vows before you as well as others. Your word says, "It is better not to vow than to make to make a vow and not fulfill it." Thank you for your help.

Scripture

"Do not be quick with your mouth, do not be hasty in the heart to utter anything before God. God is in heaven, and you are on earth, so let your words be few." (Ecclesiastes 5:6 ESV)

DAY NINETEEN

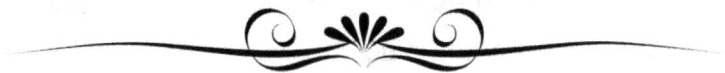

Day 19

Medical Providers Misunderstanding

"Those who sow in tears shall reap with shouts of joy!"
Psalm 126:5

When any of the medical providers wanted to do something that Tyree did not want done, I stepped in and got his wishes fulfilled. It was a struggle because sometimes medical providers do not want to hear what you have to say. They also do not always adhere to the medical directive that was signed. During his stay at one hospital, Tyree was transferred to another hospital to place a picc-line on him without my knowledge or consent. It should have been noted that they had a medical directive and copy of the Power of Attorney in his chart.

This issue made me so angry, but I did not go off the way the world says black women do. I went to the nurses' desk with tears in my eyes requesting an explanation. I requested that they pull his chart and find the Medical Directive and the Power of Attorney that shows who now makes the medical decisions on Tyree's behalf because he was no longer able to speak for himself.

The nurse located the chart with the authorization showing that I had full authority to make medical decisions for Tyree. Just when I thought everything was clear and they understood no picc-line will be placed on Tyree, a nurse came in and tried to attach one. I stood up from my chair near Tyree's bed and said, "No, this will not be happening! I did not approve this nor is it okay."

We were having to listen to them re-explain the need for the picc-line that we did not want. I patiently listened because I knew the nurse was only doing his job based on the instructions he was given. A picc-line is to ensure that Tyree would get some type of nutrients in his system because he was not able to feed himself. He did not want anyone else to feed him or be forced to eat. Giving him a picc-line was essentially force-feeding him.

My Sweet-cakes was level-headed. He was smart, sharp-minded, intelligent, clever, witty, a fixer and charming. With all that, he could not figure out how to feed himself. Therefore, he did not want me, the aides, or nurses to feed him. The picc-line was necessary according to the medical providers, but not to Tyree. He did not want to be poked or stuck anymore.

Short Prayer

Father God, you did it again. You held me up to stand on Tyree's behalf. You, oh God, gave me the words to say to the medical providers. You keep doing great things for me and Tyree. Tyree's will and Your will shall be done, and I love you for taking care both of us.

Scripture

"Blessed is the man who perseveres under trial..." (James 1:12 NIV)

DAY TWENTY

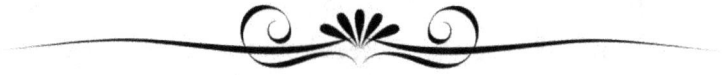

Day 20

Honor God and Tyree

"And you shall love the Lord your God with all your heart and with all your soul and with all your mind and with all your strength." (Mark 12:30 ESV)

WOW!!! THIS!!! Every day, my husband was fading away in front of my eyes and there was nothing I could do but honor his wishes along with God's guidance and instructions. Repeating and keeping the promise Tyree and I made on June 10, 2000, pushed me. The Bible says, *"Let your yes be yes and your nay be nay."* I said yes to Tyree and God helped me to keep my word. According to Matthew 5:37, *"But let your communication be, Yea, yea; Nay, nay; for whatsoever is more than these cometh of evil."* Anything other than yes cometh evil if I decided to turn from the promise I made. My yes was, "I pledge my life and love to you. In sickness and health; for richer or poorer; for better or worse until death us do part." I said these words and there is no turning back from my "yes".

I know that some of you may be wondering if I said no to this path. I did not. I did not because God told me I could not leave prior to me knowing about my Sweet-cakes' condition. We were going through some things that couples normally go through. I was looking for other places to live other than with Tyree. God said, "You cannot leave." I obeyed and then the sickness I had heard about came that I never thought would come to our house. God knew what was ahead and He knew I was the person for it. God knew Tyree would need my love to help him through this sickness that eventually took his life.

Short Prayer

Dear God, thank you for keeping me through my weakest hour. You kept me standing where I needed to stand. You helped me speak up when I needed to speak. Father God, you kept me when I wanted my flesh to operate for me. Thank you for keeping me together as I walked in your will!

Scripture

"But he said to me, "My grace is sufficient for you, for my power is made perfect in weakness." (2 Corinthians 12:9 NIV)

DAY TWENTY-ONE

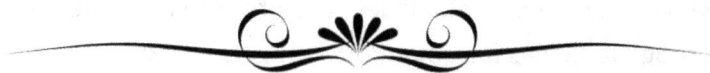

Day 21

True Commitment

"...for where you lodge, I will lodge..." (Ruth 1:16)

I committed myself to Tyree's happiness, his fulfillment, and his usefulness in God's kingdom. I made a promise to love, honor, trust, and to be with him in sickness and health, through adversity and prosperity. I promised to cleave only to him until death. The promise he made through it all was a tremendous struggle, but it was a peaceful one. It was peaceful because of the faith I have in God. God said, *"I will never leave you nor forsake you"*. Keeping that on the forefront of my mind helped me to remain at peace about God's promise that he would handle Tyree's desire.

"Be Strong and of good courage do not fear nor be afraid of them; (Dementia) *for the LORD your GOD, He is the One who goes with you. He will not leave you nor forsake you."* (Deuteronomy 31:6)

"I will keep him/her in perfect peace whose mind is stayed on me because he/she trusts me." (Isaiah 26:3)

God's word is important to me. If I didn't know it through reading, meditating, memorizing it,
I wouldn't be able to use it when I needed it. I would have turned to the ways of the world. I would have conformed to society's suggestions. I decided to listen more intensely to the voice of God through His word than people. God

kept his promise because I followed His instructions, and I was obedient to His will.

Short Prayer

Thank you, God, for never leaving me nor forsaking me. You are truly a God who loves and cares for His children. I never would have made it through this process without you being by my side. You keep your word. I am truly amazed about you. You cause me to stand in awe about how much you love us. Thank you Lord, from the bottom of my heart to the depths of my soul. Nobody can do what you do.

Scripture

"Be strong and courageous. Do not fear or be in dread of them, for it is the Lord your God who goes with you. He will not leave your or forsake you." (Deuteronomy 31:6 ESV)

DAY TWENTY-TWO

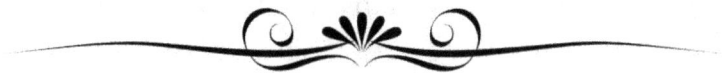

Day 22

Help Through Remembering

"Finally, be strong in the Lord and in the strength of his might." (Ephesians 6:10 KJV)

Remembering our vows and what God told me helped me to push my way through, arguments, misunderstandings, negative talking, confusion, frustration, sadness, and anger. The vows we shared to each other are filled with powerful words. God honored his promises because of my obedience and Tyree's desire to die. He did not want to live a life where he couldn't do anything for himself. He did not want to be a man that was dependent on his wife or anyone to do everything that he used to do for himself. So, he was ready be with Jesus. Can I tell you everything that he was thinking? No, I cannot. But what I can tell you is that I knew what he wanted. He wanted to die before me. He knew something I did not know. He knew that I could handle his death better than he could handle my death.

Short Prayer

Father God, you are more than awesome. Words cannot express how I feel about your goodness. Thank you for being everything I needed you to be and more. For being with me every inch of the way.

Scripture

"The Lord is my light and my salvation; who shall I fear?

the LORD is the strength of my life; of whom shall I be afraid?" (Psalm 27:1 KJV)

JANET G. MORRIS

DAY TWENTY-THREE

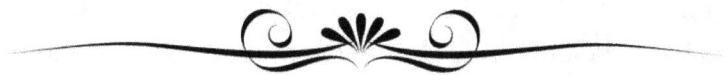

Day 23

Understanding God's Will and Tyree's Desire/Will

"Trust in the Lord with thine heart; and lean not unto thine own understanding." (Proverbs 3:5 KJV)

Although God had permitted me to pen these words to paper, I know that some people will not understand them, but it is okay. There is one thing that I want to make clear, and it is that God will do just what He said He will do. We all have choices. Tyree chose how he wanted to live, and he chose how he wanted to die. Instead of Tyree fighting against the dementia to live a little while longer, God granted Tyree's desire. Every day, I accepted Tyree's decisions and trusted God to never leave me nor forsake me.

Tyree was a champion through it all. He was my hero! He humbled himself to whatever it took to get to the place he desired; to be with his parents and Jesus. It is so fascinating how transformation takes place. He was gentle, kind, quiet, calm, and at peace. He was not as vocal as he was prior to the dementia. He didn't murmur or complain. He was being purified right in front of me. Tyree was a dark-skinned man. But his complexion began to change. His skin became soft to the touch like a newborn. The color of his skin was lightening, and a cleansing of his body was taking place in preparation to meet Jesus on the other side.

Despite all the changes that were taking place in his body, there was a twinkle in Tyree's eyes. When he opened them, there was a glassy blue color present. It was as if he could see right through to my soul. It was a warm, very comforting feeling. He was letting me know he was at peace with his decision.

Short Prayer

Dear God, help me to be at peace each day as Tyree transitions to be with Jesus. Help me to stand as your will and Tyree's desires be manifested. I can only go through this with you walking with me holding my hand.

Scripture

"Thou wilt keep him in perfect peace, whose mind is stayed on thee: because he trusteth in thee." (Isaiah 26:3 ESV)

DAY TWENTY-FOUR

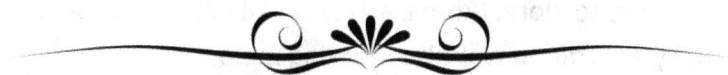

Day 24

Faith to Faith and Glory to Glory

"For this light momentary affliction is preparing for us an eternal weight of glory beyond all comparison..."
II Corinthians 4:17 (ESV)

Now that I think about it, it reminds me of a scripture in the Bible that says God is taking us from faith to faith and from glory to glory. (Romans 1:17 and II Corinthians 3:16-18). Tyree's death was also showing me our present suffering cannot compare to the glory that shall be revealed in us. (Romans 8:28) I saw the glory of God in action.

God was preparing Tyree and me for a greater glory according to His word. Tyree and I were being transformed into what God initially created us to be. We were created to worship Him. We were created to obey God's will and not our own. We were created to lean on his understanding and acknowledge him so he could direct our path (Proverbs 3:5-6). Tyree was yielding to his will as well as to the will of God. I was also yielding to the will of God. God was operating in both of us. God was giving Tyree his desires as well as transforming him into His image through death. God was transforming me into His image here on earth so the world could see that He is God.

God was preparing me for things to come, things I had no idea would transpire after Tyree's death: the loss of my health; the loss of companionship; the loss of our house; the loss of income; the loss of friends and family members. The glory of God will still shine through it all. God's glory will shine through me, through my attitude, my actions, my walk, and my talk. God did it.

Short Prayer

Oh my God, you are so AWESOME. How you made us shine through it all is simply amazing! You show up every time. Thank you! Thank You! Thank You! Thank You!

Scripture

"...but we also glory in our sufferings, because we know that suffering produces perseverance, perseverance, character; and character hope." (Romans 5: 3b-5 NIV)

DAY TWENTY-FIVE

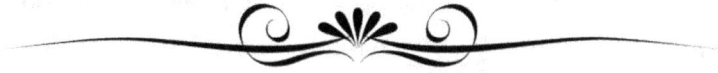

Day 25

Suffering Through

"...knowing that he who raised the Lord Jesus will raise us also with Jesus and bring us with you in his presence."
(2 Corinthians 4:14 ESV)

Through all his suffering and his forgetting, Tyree did not forget me or my youngest son Mon. During his death journey, Tyree kept asking me, "Where is Mon?" He asked Mon to do his eulogy, which he did and did a great job, despite it being his first time doing a eulogy. I applaud him for stepping in where he was asked. It took courage and faith in God to do what Tyree requested. Tyree wanted to be assured that all his requests were being met. He called for Mon a lot during his last moments on earth. (Side note: Zephaniah I, my daughter-in-law Shekeyva (not Zephaniah I's wife), the hospice nurse, and I were there when he died. It was just like God said it would be... peaceful.

I can imagine that Tyree was filled with the joy of the Lord because if he never got everything he wanted while here on earth, he was most definitely getting it now. He got to go home to be with the Lord. It was his choice, his right, his will, and his desire to die before me. He did it graciously. I love him for that.

For me, life will still go on with the help of the Lord.

Short Prayer

God, you are more than enough. You have truly shown yourself mighty through this struggle. That is why we both are winning. You made it all possible because of your love for us. I thank you from the bottom of my heart to the depths of my soul.

Scripture

"Oh give thanks to the Lord, for He is good; for his steadfast love endures forever!" (I Chronicles 16:34 KJV)

DAY TWENTY-SIX

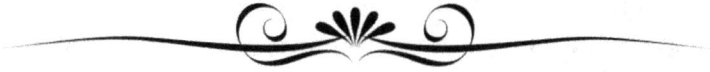

Day 26

The Purification

"Create in me a clean heart, O god and renew a right spirit within me. Cast me not away from thy presence; and take not thy Holy Spirit from me". (Psalm 51: 10-11ESV)

Understanding the cleansing that was going on through me during this death journey is so insightful. It caused me, someone who considers herself to be a child of God, to reflect on my life. An evaluation was taking place, not of Tyree but of me, the person who refused to follow the world's ways but wanted to uphold her vows.

"You burn just a little more flesh. You die just a little more while God is increasing in you for you to do greater. You walk out the love of God." (Genesis Marie, my granddaughter)

The steadfast love of God is so unexplainable to the carnal mind. Experiencing God's love can be so overwhelming that it makes you fall to your knees and worship Him. It brings tears to your eyes, tears of joy. There is nothing that can compare to the steadfast love of God. According to Christianty201.wordpress.com, steadfast love is mentioned 196 times in the Old Testament, 127 times in the Psalms alone.

God's love is not going anywhere. It is always present and ready to hug you, kiss you, hold you, care for you, forgive you, rebuke you, and give you chances to get it right.

STRUGGLING AND WINNING

"Because of His great love we are not consumed, for his compassions never fail." (Lamentations 3:22 NIV)

During Tyree's death journey, I was dying daily and being purified. God was cleansing me from all selfish things, jealousy, hatred, and anger within me. God was pushing Himself out of me for the world to see.

God allowed me the opportunity to evaluate my life, my thoughts, my words, and my love for Tyree. How was I living my life as I proclaimed the Gospel of Jesus Christ? Was my life truly exemplifying Christ-like characteristics? How did the world see me as a minister of God? How did they see my love for Tyree? How did the world see me as a wife? How did the world see me as a mother? How did the world see me as an individual? How did God see me? How did I see myself? Was I living to please man or God?

All these things unfolded on my journey of dying to self. Death hurts. It's very painful to let go of something or someone you love, something or someone you do not believe you can live without. It is not that I thought I could not live without Tyree; I just never thought about him dying that soon into our marriage. I knew he had some ailments, but I never thought dementia would be added to the equation.

Therefore, I began to live a life of love, compassion, and concern, a life of meekness and kindness. It was not my will, but God's will and Tyree's choice to die in peace and die before me. Things began to transpire in a way that would seem foolish to others, but it made sense to me because God was talking to me. The peace came when I began looking at our finances and Tyree's medical care cost. God touches the hearts of the people and entities that you turn to for help. I reported all our income and expenses, down to how many vehicles we owned and how much our insurance policies were. To this today, I do not know why they need to know the amount of our insurance policies. I received a letter of approval for Tyree stating that they were only going to use Tyree's income. My God!!! PEACE!!! GOD IS AWESOME!

Short Prayer

Lord God Almighty, you keep proving yourself to me over and over. You do not change. You stand by your word. Your word doesn't return void. You are not a God that would lie neither a son of man who must repent. Thank you for standing by your word.

Scripture

"Jesus Christ the same yesterday and today and forever." (Hebrews 13: 8 ESV)

DAY TWENTY-SEVEN

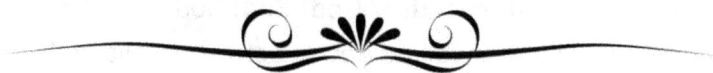

Day 27

Believing and Erasing the Doubts

"...I do believe; help me overcome my unbelief!"
(Mark 9:24 NIV)

My life changed. I just began to believe even more of what God said to me in August 2011. My prayers began to reflect the will of God. God, how do I handle this? God, with whom do I discuss this? God! God! God! God, I cannot handle this if you do not go before me and with me. I need you Jesus. I cannot make it or do it without you. HELP ME JESUS!!!

Sometimes, my prayer would be a whisper, a thought, or one sentence... Lord, help me! Whether I'd scream with tears in my eyes, kneel, walk, or drive, I had to build my faith so I could erase doubt. Everything I did, everywhere I went, I just wanted to be in the will of God.

Short Prayer

You were there all the time waiting patiently in line. God, thank you for waiting on me. Thank you for giving me multiple chances to recognize that you are the Lord. Thank you for loving me so much that I cannot articulate how much I appreciate you.

Scripture

"Now faith is the substance of things hoped for and the evidence of things not seen." (Hebrews 11:1 KJV)

DAY TWENTY-EIGHT

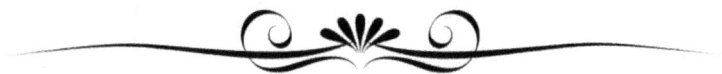

Day 28

Words

"Death and life are in the power of the tongue…"
Proverbs 18:21 (ESV)

I noticed the words that were coming out of my mouth and how they influenced how I handled Tyree's requests and decisions. He was adamant about his decision despite doctors and nurses trying to convince him to fight. I had to do what Tyree wanted and not what I thought or desperately wanted.

I wanted him to live for a long time, if possible. I wanted him to accept at-home medical care with the help of outside caregivers. I wanted him to exercise his brain by doing puzzles like he used to love to do. I wanted him to continue to play dominos and go on walks with me holding my hand while laughing. I wanted him to do at-home therapy recommended by his doctor. I wanted him to get out of bed even if I or the caregiver had to assist him. I wanted… but Tyree did not want any of these things. He wanted to lay there and not be bothered. He wanted what he wanted, and he was not going to change his mind.

This was Tyree's final decision. Therefore, my words had to reflect his wishes, desires, decisions, and requests, not anyone else's. He was determined.

Determined: having a firm decision and being resolved not to change it. (adjective)

(Verb) cause (something) to occur in a particular way; be the deceive factor in. (bing.com)

Short Prayer

Father God, you are holy and faithful. You are the Great I Am. You allowed Tyree's wishes to go forth. You helped me to remain focused on you and Tyree. There is no other way I could have done this. Thank you, God, for giving me the wisdom to recognize the words that were proceeding out of my mouth.

Scripture

"Looking unto Jesus the author and finisher of our faith…" (Hebrews 12:2 KJV)

DAY TWENTY-NINE

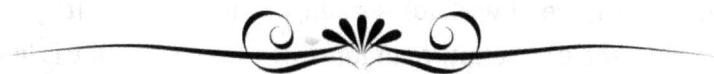

Day 29

Starting Over

"Do not boast about tomorrow, for you do not know what a day may bring." (Proverbs 27:1 ESV)

Starting over after Tyree's death was a struggle. There is an emptiness and loneliness that comes along with being alone. Life, as you thought, is no longer. He was here and now he is gone. It was not sudden, but it felt like it. It reminds me of a scripture in James 4:14 that says life is like a vapor. We are here and then we are gone. It is like a mist from a teapot. If you turn the fire off under the teapot, the mist slowly disappears. Tyree disappeared from my life. Now what? Despite the pain, the grief, and the mourning, life goes on with Jesus on the journey with me.

Yes, Jesus helped through it all. He comforted me, encouraged me, strengthened me, and kept me focused on Him. Why would he tell me about Tyree's death if he was not going to guide me all the way? What is so amazing is that he did not have to tell me. I am forever grateful that He chose to tell me, to give me a warning of what was going to happen ahead of time. It showed me that I have favor with God, just like David was an apple of God's eye. (Psalm 17:8)

Short Prayer

Father God, thank you for giving me a favor I did not deserve to allow me the opportunity to prepare for Tyree's death. It is so amazing and awesome to me. You are so loving and caring. I thank you from the bottom of my heart and to the depths of my soul. You are truly an Awesome God.

Scripture

"Blessed are they that mourn for they shall be comforted." (Matthew 5:4 KJV)

DAY THIRTY

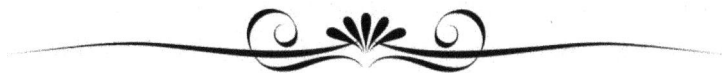

Day 30

Choices

"...I have set before you, life and death, blessing and the curse: therefore, choose life, that you and your offspring may live..." (Deuteronomy 30:19 ESV)

I have been taught all my life that everyone has a choice. We all have free will to pick and choose what we want in life or out of life. The choice that Tyree made was shocking to me when we initially discussed it. I cannot remember why we discussed death so much during our nine years of marriage. I still do not know why.

I never thought about who would or should die first. I remember asking him, "How do you know you would not be able to go on living if I died first?" He responded, "I know what I want." Tyree saw something that God knew, and I did not see or know. Tyree knew I would be okay even if it did not look or seem like it to me.

Short Prayer

God almighty, you helped me to be okay. Father God, you helped me to not lose my mind. You strengthen me every step of the way. I give your name the glory, and I praise your holy name. Thank you!

Scripture

"The Lord is thy keeper; The LORD is thy shade upon thy right hand." (Psalm 121:5 KJV)

DAY THIRTY-ONE

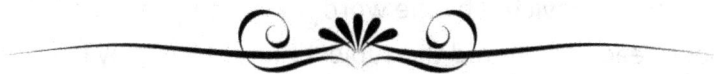

Day 31

Why Get Married?

"...If anyone would come after me, let him deny himself and take up his cross and follow me." (Matthew 16:24 ESV)

I married Tyree following a broken engagement with another man. My desire to be married was mostly based on my belief that sex should be reserved for marriage. I had been convicted by the word of God because I had been teaching around the subject but not living by it.

In the beginning, I used to believe I was saved—that is, until I went through some struggles I tried to fix on my own. I was not praying appropriately to God to fix it. Actually, I did not pray at all. I went through life trying to work it out on my own. I cannot say what I was thinking. I was simply living without considering the costs or consequences of my decisions, or how they would affect me, my children, and my family.

I died along with Tyree. There was no more selfish motive, no more wanting to leave Tyree; only love reigned at this moment. The glory of God was revealed within us. *"Our present suffering cannot be compared to the glory that shall be revealed in us."* (Romans 8:28) There was no escaping this suffering. I had to stay the course with Jesus on my side guiding me all the way. He was my helper, my sustainer; my light, and my salvation. *"The Lord is my light and my salvation; whom shall, I fear? The Lord is the stronghold of my life; of whom shall I be afraid?"* (Psalm 27:1 ESV).

I am more than a conqueror. Greater is He that is in me than he that is in the world. Jesus helped me through the process. So, here I am going through it once again. I am dealing with my own sickness/disease. I remember how Jesus was with me during Tyree's sickness/disease then death. This time, I know what God can do. Since I know what God is capable of, it helps me to stay focus on the healer that He is. I have learned to accept the way He wants to heal me on this side or on the other side.

The pain that I deal with within my body daily is no joke. No one can relate to the type of pain that I experience, not even the doctors. The pain can be so excruciating that all I can say is, "Jesus! Jesus!" until the pain subsides. One minute of severe pain can seem like 15-20 minutes.

Sometimes, the pain medication, the pain patches, heating pad, and pain gel don't work. I pray for relief and remain calm as Jesus does His work on me. Once, when I was in pain, I felt Jesus kneeling at my feet holding my hand helping me to relax as the pain left my body. I was in awe of how much He loves and cares for me. "Be still and know that I am God." (Psalm 46:10)

Slow down and feel my presence. Slow down and hear my voice. Slow down and feel my touch. You are busy trying to do it yourself. Let me do what I do. You are trying too hard and still not getting anywhere. Let me do it and it will be done. It will be completed. The glory will be revealed in you; but the glory that is being revealed in you is my glory; the glory that the world needs to see. "For I reckon that the sufferings of this present time are not worthy to be compared with the glory which shall be revealed in us." (Romans 8:18 KJV)

Short Prayer

Father God, creator of the Heavens and the Earth. You alone are God. No one can take your place and I am grateful for that. I am grateful for all things that you have allowed to transpire in my life to show me your faithfulness, your mercy, and grace toward Tyree and I. You are extremely AMAZING!

Scripture

"And we know that for those who love God all things to work together for the good, for those who are called according to his purpose. (Romans 8:28 ESV)

DAY THIRTY-TWO

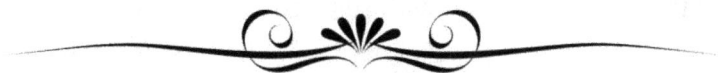

Day 32

Memories

"But Mary treasured up all these things, pondering them in her heart." (Luke 2:19 ESV)

When I say Tyree was my protector, I mean it. Tyree would carry a switchblade to church in his pocket. I was not aware of this until an incident occurred at church where he thought I was upset with someone. He ran toward me with his hand in his pocket asking, "What is going on?" I asked, "Why do you have your hand in your pocket?" He showed me the switchblade. I told him not to pull that knife out, everything is okay, and he backed off. He did not go anywhere without taking his switchblade.

One time we were preparing dinner. He was outside getting the grill ready, and I was inside preparing the vegetables and salad. I put a round peppermint in my mouth and it got lodged in my throat. I couldn't say anything. I ran outside and Tyree looked up and immediately ran to me. He hit me in the middle of my back and the peppermint went flying out of my mouth. He then grabbed me and held me tightly. I did not have to say a word. He ran to me and rescued me. Thank you, Jesus.

When we went shopping together, he would walk behind me. One day, I asked him why. He just smiled. So, another day, I decided to walk side-by-side with him and when I stopped to look at something, he waited so he could walk behind me. I found out that he liked the way I walk.

One time, he noticed I was contemplating buying an outfit. I decided not to get it and when I got to the cashier with the items I wanted to purchase, he brought the other outfit to the register and purchase it as well. He loved buying me clothes and shoes.

I miss him. I wrote a poem called, "Why Visit the Grave?"

December 22, 2015

Why Visit the Grave?

He cannot hear me!
The flowers he cannot smell.
My present flowers, he is not aware?
The body lying there has no senses, touch, smell, see, hear, taste.
The body cannot respond to any of my actions nor respond when I talk or wipe away my tears.
Why visit the grave?

Because there is comfort
Because there is peace
Because just the thought of remembering brings some type of relief from the pressure you feel deep within
For me, is that really relief?
I go to the grave for me...not him because his soul is not there.

What relief? An unexplained pressure, an unexplained desire
Even though you know there will be no response from the one you hold dear.

He lay sleep in the grave without a response that will
comfort you or bring you relief.
But you still feel something even that is better than
nothing.
Is that truly relief?
Is it in my mind? So, I go to the grave.
But why go to the grave?

It is not out of guilt.
Because he knows, he knew that I loved him.
I have nothing to prove.
So why go to the grave?

His spirit is not there; that is what made him exist.
He cannot kiss me.
He cannot hug me.
He cannot talk to me.
He cannot give me that familiar sexy smile.
So, why do I go to the grave?
It is a satisfaction in knowing that I really loved him, and I
miss him?
The grave is a place I can spend time remembering...

The grave is a place of rest for the body to turn back to
dust according to the word of God.
*"In the sweat of thy face shalt thou eat bread, till the
return unto the ground, for out of it were you taken; for
dust you are dust, and to dust you shall return.* (Genesis
3:19 ESV)
Your existence on Earth is no more.
If you are now dust, why do I continue to go to the grave?
Why go to the grave when evidence says you are dust?
Your existence has ceased to be.
The very idea of talking to you makes no sense.

The idea of taking flowers to your place of rest to be thrown away makes no sense.
Yet, I find myself going to the grave.

Sometimes I feel as though you are here.
It is as if I can reach out and touch you...because what I feel/sense is real.
It is pulling me to go back in time to see what occurred before you left this earth.
It pulls me to a place where you existed in my life (memories).
Memories bring joy, sadness, happiness, heartache, pain, tears...soon no more tears of sadness but tears of joy, to smiles, to laughter (repeating without notice) the pain that comes with grief.

Why visit the grave where your body lay or used to lay because now it is dust or is it?
How long does it take for a body to turn back to dust?
"For the grave cannot praise thee, death cannot celebrate thee: they that go down into the pit cannot hope for thy truth." (Isaiah 38:18 KJV)
There is no life in the grave.
So why visit the grave?

"What profit is there in my blood, if I go down to the pit? Shall the dust praise thee? Shall it declare thy truth?" (Psalm 30:9 KJV)
"For in death there is no remembrance of thee: in the grave who shall give thee thanks? (Psalm 6:5 KJV)
If there is no life at this place of rest,
Why does it pull me back to a place where life does not exist?
Why do I visit the grave?

Is it for solitude?
He cannot respond to how I act or what I say...
This question continues to linger in my mind.
Maybe there is no answer to this question that visits me
on occasion, that will satisfy me.
My soul still longs for your presence, your existence. You
were here and now you are there.
Nothing will happen until Jesus' return.
You will rise because of your belief in Him.
*"For the Lord himself will descend from heaven with a
shout, with the voice of an archangel, and with the trump
of God: and the dead in Christ will rise first. Then who are
alive and remain shall be caught up together with them in
the clouds, to meet the Lord in the air: and so, shall we
ever be with the Lord."* (1 Thessalonians 4:16-17 KJV)

God will bring you to Jesus first, then me if Jesus returns
before I die. If not, we will rise up together. Either way, we
will meet again...but not at the grave.

Visit: Go to see and spend time with (someone) socially.
(Merriam Webster)
Greek definition episkeptomai/episkopos, which is
rendered "overseer" In Acts 20:28. Thayer, the great Greek
lexicographer, defines the word, "to look upon or after, to
inspect, examine with the eyes to look upon in order to
help or benefit." (truthmagazine.com)
The question still remains, Why visit the grave, when I
know you are not there?

WHY? WHY? WHY? WHY? WHY?

Short Prayer

Father God, going to the grave doesn't make sense to me right now. I am aware, based on your word, that he is not there because his soul is with you. Yet, there is a yearning to go and visit Tyree's grave. I know my comfort comes from not going to the grave. God, I need you to help me do what is right in your sight. I desire to be in your will. I also do not want to rely on Tyree's gravesite to bring me hope.

Scripture

"I will praise the LORD, who counsels me, even at night my hear instructs me." (Psalm 5:8 NIV)

JANET G. MORRIS

DAY THIRTY-THREE

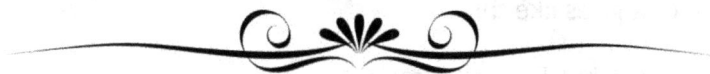

Day 33

A Closer Walk with God

"...The Lord, before whom I walk [habitually and obediently], will send His angel with you to make your journey successful..." (Genesis 24:40 AMP)

One day I was talking to God and a song Tyree used to sing at church... "Just a Closer Walk with Thee"... came to my mind. It goes like this:

I am weak but Thou art strong
Jesus keep me from all wrong
I'll be satisfied as long
As I walk, let me walk close to Thee

Just a closer walk with Thee
Grant it, Jesus, is my plea
Daily walking close to Thee
Let it be, dear Lord, let it be

When my feeble life is o'er
Time for me will be no more
Guide me gently, safely o'er
To Thy kingdom's shore, to Thy shore

Just a closer walk with Thee
Grant it, Jesus, is my plea
Daily walking close to Thee
Let it be, dear Lord, let it be

This song was Tyree's desire to walk closer with Jesus. He wanted to have the opportunity to be in the presence of the Lord the way he chose to be. I am so proud of him. He died strong. He died with dignity. He died peacefully. His choice, and no one else's.

Short Prayer

Lord, how majestic is your name in the all the earth. There is none like you. You're such an amazing God. You know exactly what I need and how I would react toward Tyree's death, and you made it joyful and peaceful.

Scripture

"I have set the Lord always before me; Because He is my right hand I shall not be moved." (Psalm 16:8 NKJV)

JANET G. MORRIS

DAY THIRTY-FOUR

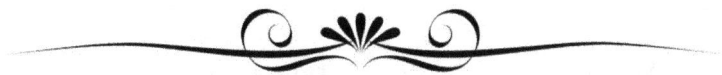

Day 34

Knowing God Through the Struggle

"For God so loved the world..." (John 3:16 KJV)

Through the struggle, I recognized that God really loves me. Despite my evil ways, God still loves me. He showed me so much love during this struggle. Words in the English dictionary cannot fully describe the love that God has for us, for me.

According to the word of God, his love is steadfast.

"Oh, give thanks to the Lord, for he is good; for his steadfast love endures forever." (Psalm 118:1 ESV)

Steadfast: resolutely or dutifully firm and unwavering. (Dictionary.com)

Biblically Merriam-Webster

Steadfast: 1a: firmly fixed in place: immovable.

As I go through this struggle of Tyree physical death and my death to self, I realize just how much love God has for me. Frist of all, He did not have to tell me that Tyree's condition would lead to death. God could have kept that information to himself and allowed me to deal with it when it happened. God loves me so much that he told me. He guided me through the process and the death. He never left me to my own devices, ideas, strategies, and or thoughts. God provided me everything I needed to go through Tyree's sickness, his family, my family, and his death. It was well orchestrated.

God showed up in a way that caused me to stand in AWE of his love, mercy, and grace. God is so God! He is more than I can express. I want to shout with joy when I think about the goodness of God in my life. His love is truly overwhelming.

God's love brings me tears of joy, a smile on my face, and confidence in knowing the love He has for me. His love is not just for me; he loves the whole world. His love never runs out. Even if I stopped worshipping Him, He would still love me, but I cannot stop loving God. He is so faithful. He keeps His word. He showed me His word throughout my struggle, and continues to show Himself through His word. "There is nothing my God cannot do!"

Short Prayer

Father God, creator of all things, I love you because you have shown me what love looks like. I thought I knew but you showed me real love. Thank you for looking at me and showing me me.

Scripture

"Love is patient and kind; love does not envy or boast; it is not arrogant or rude. It does not insist on its own way; it is not irritable or resentful;" (I Cor. 13:4-5 ESV)

DAY THIRTY-FIVE

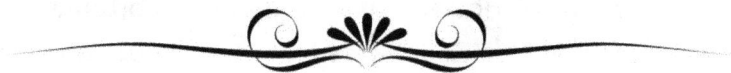

Day 35

Taking God with you through the Struggle

"Trust in the Lord with thy heart and lean not unto thine own understanding…" (Proverbs 3:5-6 KJV)

I heard the voice of God speaking to me. It took God talking to me three times before I realized He was speaking to me. I had to realize that Tyree's condition was out of my control. However, it was also my opportunity to walk in the direction God planned for me and put my trust in Him. God's desire is for me to allow His presence to be present in everything that I do.

Psalm 46:10 (KJV) *"Be still and know that I am God; I will be exalted among the heathen, I will be exalted in the earth."* Through this incident, I was able to be still and recognize what God doing in my life, both now and in the future.

I no longer had the distraction of giving medical updates to people who did not believe the medical report given. I did not have to listen to people talk about me and my children after listening to them for so many years. It was somewhat of a relief, but at the same time, it wasn't. I did not understand why some people did not believe the medical report I was giving them from Tyree's doctors. With each report of his condition getting worse, it was giving them the opportunity to spend more time with him instead of using me as a punching bag.

It is possible that they did not see it that way. They were not privy to what God told me. I was not able to share with them what God had said and the instructions he had given me, which was a struggle. This is where I learned the true meaning of the scripture, *"The natural person does not accept the things of the Spirit of God, for they are folly to him, and he is not able to understand them because they are spiritually discerned."* (2 Corinthians 2:14 ESV)

God said, *"Lo I am with you always even unto the ends of the earth."* There was something inside of me that caused me to push toward God more and more. It caused me to seek God regarding everything that occurred in my life. I am still leaning on Him. Do I always get it right? No, but I am striving every day to have a closer walk with God, better than I did the day before. My relationship with God is nowhere close to how it used to be.

Psalm 46 begins with: *"God is our refuge and strength, a very present help in trouble..."* Whatever the danger, God is my refuge, and he will give me the strength to endure the struggle and the war.

Short Prayer

Heavenly Father, thank you for strengthening me through the weakest time of this journey. Thank you for keeping me each time I was about to fall, placing my foot on solid ground to continue this journey.

Scripture

"But the Helper, the Holy Spirit, whom the Father will send in my name, he will teach you all things and bring to your remembrance all that I have said to you. (John 14:26 ESV)

DAY THIRTY-SIX

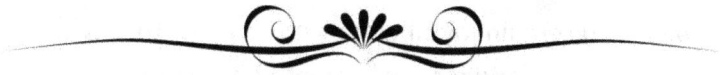

Day 36

Try to Remain Joyful

"Count it all joy, my brothers, when you meet trials of various kinds... the test of your faith produces steadfastness..." (James 1:2-3 ESV)

"...My grace is sufficient for thee: for my power is made perfect in weakness." (2 Corinthians 12:9 ESV)

How do you remain joyful when you're going through heartache, pain, and disappointment? It is very hard. It's a struggle to remain focused on where your strength comes from. Therefore, you must press your way through the negative thoughts and words that challenge your joy.

But how can you do this alone? How can you handle all the pressure of so many things going on at the same time? How do you navigate losing relationships at the same time you are dealing with issues that are beyond your control? This pressure is beyond anything you could imagine. But when it's over, you realize that God was with you through it all. You get a better understanding of why you really need God in your life, completely and totally.

This experience has made me take a closer look at the scriptures. The one stated above has been proven to me repeatedly. I lived it through this death journey, and I am living now through my sickness/disease. It is truly amazing how God shows you that His strength is made perfect when you are weak. I noticed the above noted scripture on days when I felt weak in my physical body, but my spirit would be willing.

It also reminds me of Matthew 26:41 which says, *"...the spirit is indeed willing, but the flesh is weak."* This is when Jesus asked Peter, James, and John to go with him to the Garden of Gethsemane to watch and pray. They fell asleep each time Jesus prayed. To me, it feels like an outer body experience. My physical being is watching my spiritual being do the things my physical being couldn't. My spiritually being (Jesus) knows it must be done and so He helps me get it done.

Short Prayer

Thank you, heavenly Father, for making your strength perfect in me when I am weak. I would not have been able to do what you instructed me to do on this journey to purification.

Scripture

"Blessed are the pure in heart, for they shall see God." (Matthew 5:8 ESV)

DAY THIRTY-SEVEN

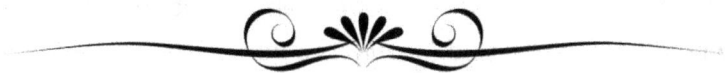

Day 37

"The Pressures of Life"

"Fear not for I am with you; be not dismayed...I will uphold you with my righteous right hand." (Isaiah 41:10; KJV)

As noted on day 36, I was trying to remain joyful throughout the journey of death... not only mine, but Tyree's as well. I was reminded that God will uphold me with his righteous right hand because he told me what would happen. He told me what to do and say, so that meant He would not allow my joy to dwindle. He would be right there to remind me who He is to me.

If I lean on him with each step, He will not leave me nor forsake me. He will keep His promise to remain with me throughout this process. He will be the strength I need to make it through everything that transpires. He would be the one to take the wheel of decisions. He did all of that and more. He brought forth love, joy, and peace. He kept His word, He showed His word, and He worked His word through me.

There were times I screamed out loud and hit the wall because the pressure felt like it was too much to deal with, but I never forgot what God said. When I cried, I could feel God's hands holding me and whispering scriptures in my ear to help me endure the pain of death, lost relationships, life after Tyree's death, and life of being totally committed to God.

Being aware of God's presence through it all helped me to withstand the storms of life. It helped to build my focus and strength. It helped me to build my belief in God, which produced a more intimate relationship with Him.

Short Prayer

Thank you, God, for manifesting your words throughout the process. Thank you for allowing me the opportunity to have a closer relationship with you and to know you better than I was allowing myself. You are truly amazing. God, you're more than that.

Scripture

"The Lord is my light and my salvation: whom shall, I fear? The Lord is the strength of my life; of whom shall I be afraid?" (Psalm 27:1; KJV)

JANET G. MORRIS

DAY THIRTY-EIGHT

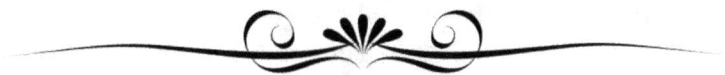

Day 38

Staying Focused on God

"I will lift my eyes unto the hills...My help comes from the Lord...He will not allow your foot to slip;"
(Psalm 121: 1-3; AMP)

What kept me focused on God? I did not know exactly how everything would play out for me. Would I lose what God was trying to do in me and through me? How would I come out on the other side? The other side showed me exactly how I should always look toward God.

One of my favorite scriptures is Proverbs 3:5-6, *"Trust in the Lord with all thine heart, and lean not unto thine own understanding. In all thy ways acknowledge him, and he shall direct thy paths."* (KJV) I didn't always practice this scripture, but now I do. It took going through my death journey to get to this place of relying on God no matter what.

During the path of death and purification, I began to see just how much I needed to call on the name of the Lord. Not to say that I didn't previously, but I was not calling on Him like it is stated in Proverbs 3:5-6. Prior to my experience, I discussed with others what I was going through to see what they had to say.

You see, in the scripture, it did not instruct me to lean on others for directions. It says, "Trust in the Lord and lean not on your own understanding." That lets me know that my trust was not completely in the Lord God Almighty. I had to revisit the scripture, recite it, meditate on it, and apply it. And as I did, my mind became clear, and my vision was renewed.

I had to be committed to reading the scriptures, reciting the scriptures, meditating on the scriptures, and applying the scriptures daily, not just when I felt I needed the Lord. What do I do now that I have pushed to this place in God? How do I respond to this? I asked myself questions like "What did God say about this?" and "What does God's word say about that?"

For me to focus on God completely, I had to drown out the noise. Sometimes, I attempted to choke out the noise with music, prayer, scriptures (read aloud), and hollering out the words of God from memory. I also anointed myself and my house with oil. (This needs to be a teaching.)

Side note: The Holy Spirit is amazing because He will teach all things and bring to your remembrance the scriptures you have meditated on. (John 14:26)

Today, I can share that my focus on God is stronger than it was when the struggle and trials began. I can proudly say that God stepped in every time because I applied Proverbs 3:5-8. There are other passages of scriptures that I applied, but it will take several books for me to share them all with you.

Short Prayer

Father God, I appreciate you more than words can express. I am who I am because of you. I made it through because of you and you are still holding me up. Thank you, God, from the bottom of my heart to the depth of my soul.

Scripture

"But when the Father sends the Advocate as my representative-that is, the Holy Spirit-he will teach you everything and will remind you of everything I have told you." (John 14:26; NLT)

DAY THIRTY-NINE

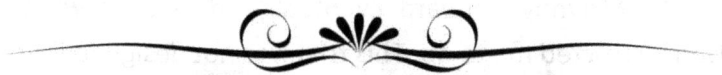

Day 39

"Staying in the Will of God"

"Seek ye first the kingdom of God, and his righteousness, and all these things shall be." (KJV)

Seeking God's will with each step and decision really was a struggle. I made many decisions after discussing things with people, talking to God, and combining what I thought was best to move forward. Eventually, I did exactly what God instructed me to do. This trial was not designed for me to discuss things with others before God gave me the release. My only option was to completely depend on God.

Being in a place of total dependency on God caused me to be silent and to choose my words carefully when I did speak. *"Death and life are in the power of the tongue and they that love it shall eat the fruit thereof."* (Proverbs 18:21) My conversation changed. I closely monitored what came out of my mouth. It pushed me to ask people about what was going on with them. I wanted to do whatever I could do to encourage others and not focus on my issues.

I sent out encouragement cards. As I reached out to others, I began to feel closer to God. That was important as I still faced so many unknown situations. I knew that Tyree's disease was going to lead to death but not knowing when is what pushed me to want to be in God's presence. *"To walk in the spirit and not fulfill the lust of the flesh"* (Galatians 5:16).

I did not always walk in the spirit. I tried to figure out things on my own or with others' opinions. Even though I knew the scriptures, I still relied on my own understanding and the world, instead of the one who created the world. I called on God after the fact, after screwing things up. After traveling the road of disappointments, I would cry out to the Lord for help. What I thought would break me made me a better person, a stronger servant of the Lord.

I am so glad I was given the opportunity to walk this path with God on my side. He knew I was good enough when I thought I wasn't. God loved me enough to share this secret of death with only me and walked right along with me. It was so amazing to be chosen by God.

Knowing how much God loves me helped me to deal with the outcome. He helped me to understand his sovereignty. He helped me to rely on him and trust him in all things. He continues to remind me of Jeremiah 29:11 - *"For I know the thoughts that I think toward you, saith the LORD, thoughts of peace, and not of evil, to give you an expected end."* (KJV)

There is nothing that God does not know. There is nothing that He cannot do. There is no place where He is not. I was walking around like God did not know my life in its totality. I knew, but I did not recognize or accept that He is the all-knowing God. I was taught this in scriptures, but my maturity level in Christ was on a very low scale. I had to learn to apply the scriptures, talk about the scriptures, meditate on the scriptures, and give God's words back to

Him.

As I did, my relationship with God changed, which led to my relationships with myself and others changing, too. Love was stronger. The love for God, love for myself, love for Tyree, and love for my neighbor. My relationship with God continues to change for the better. I am fixing my eyes and ears on God, which makes things better through the struggles, trials, and tribulation.

Short Prayer

Father God, you are AWESOME. You are more than AWESOME. You are faithful to me and all your creations. I thank you for all you have and are doing in my life. Without you, I would not have made it to the other side with my light shining bright.

Scripture

"Ye are the light of the world. A city that is set on an hill cannot be hid." (Matthew 5:14 KJV)

DAY FORTY

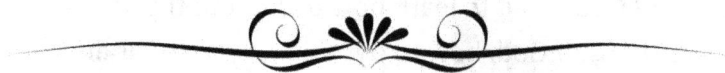

Day 40

Allowing the process to show you, You

"Examine yourselves, whether ye be in the faith; prove your own selves. Know ye not your own selves, how that Jesus Christ is in you, except ye be reprobates?"
2 Corinthians 13:5

This was a time for me to examine myself according to the Word of God. I had to learn how to react to the instructions of God, how to put aside my agendas and plans and be more committed to the will of God and Tyree's will. I had to grow to a place of acceptance. It took a lot of examining. I knew that I did not want to go against the will of God. I also knew I had to keep the covenant I made with Tyree on our wedding day. I promised him that I would be there for him, and I would do my best to fulfill his desires, even though it was hard to do.

During that examination period, I found that my relationship with God was stronger than I imagined. At the same time, I realized that God really cared for me, and that God is more than I can imagine. The Bible says that God can do even more than I can imagine. *"...according to the power that worketh in (me) us..."* (*Ephesians 3:20*)

I found out that God works in me based on the power that is within me, the power that God put in me when he breathed the breath of life in me, and I became a living soul. (Genesis 1:26) The Bible declares that God did not give us the spirit of fear. God gave us power, love, and a sound mind. *(2 Timothy 1: 6)* I could not allow fear to take me on a different path. I had to be persistent with the word of God during my examination, death journey and purification process. I was determined not to allow anything to take me off course. This examination and purification process pushed me to have a closer relationship with God. As I examined my motives during the purification and Tyree's death, I began to see myself and others through God's eyes. I had been seeing only what I wanted to see and ignored what others might be experiencing. It also caused me to look at all people as God's precious creation, not just some people.

My self-examination revealed that I was struggling with the news that Tyree's condition would worsen and that it would lead to death rather than recovery. My prayers would not be to heal Tyree on earth, but to assist him in the process of dying, to assist him in reaching the goal he had set for himself, which was to live eternally with Jesus. Tyree would tell me how much he missed his father and mother. He would talk about seeing them sitting on his bed and Jesus at the foot of his bed.

I had to be in the present, but also reflect on the past while considering the future. Some of the choices I made were not in the will of God. Romans 8:28 says, *"And we know that all things work together for good to them who love God, to them who are the called according to his purpose."* I stand in AWE of God's love for me.

I contemplated continuing with my bachelor's degree after being out of school for 34 years. How can I attend college and take care of Tyree or be at the hospital to ensure that the doctors and nurses were following his wishes? Should I continue even though I knew it was stressful trying to keep everything together? The stress was so overwhelming that it became hard for me to study, read, complete assignments, and keep track of the doctors and nurses. I had a conversation with God, then the school. I was given time off from school to put my focus on Tyree's care.

Short Prayer

Thank you, God, for being who you are in my life, for showing up each time I needed you. I truly appreciate you for all the things you do and continue to do. You're a Sovereign God.

Scripture

"Be still and know that I am God; I will be exalted among the nations, I will be exalted in the earth!" (Psalm 46:10 ESV)

DAY FORTY-ONE

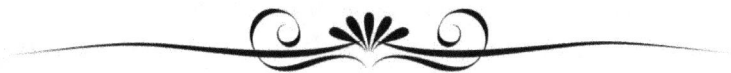

Day 41

Walking through the Death Valley"

"Even when I walk through the darkest valley, I will not be afraid, for you are close beside me." (Psalm 23:4)

This scripture spoke to me during Tyree's death. I have known this scripture for over 50 years, and I did not connect to it until then. Even though there had been several deaths in my family, this was different; it was someone I had made a pledge to. This was the second time I made a pledge like this. I was determined to get it right this time. The thought of leaving Tyree did not enter my mind, thanks to God putting a stop to the negative thoughts flooding my mind 4-5 years prior to Tyree's diagnosis with dementia. We pledged to each other to be there until death takes us away. We did it! Hallelujah!!!

Walking through this dark valley was better than I thought it would be. I realized that these trials did not come to make me fall; they came to strengthen me. They came to give me a chance to live out the vows I made to Tyree because I did not fulfill the same vows with my previous husband. I got to experience what it looks and feels like to love until death and to walk through the hurt and pain of death with God by my side every step of the way.

God said, "I will never leave you nor forsake you." God did not allow me to suffer alone. He did not reveal to me Tyree's death then leave me to deal with it on my own. He let me know that his glory would be revealed. Paul wrote in Romans 8:18, *"I consider that our present sufferings are not worth comparing with the glory that will be revealed in us."* Tyree's death, my death journey/purification was revealing the glory of God. Every word of this scripture manifested this shadow of death. I could put my trust in God and know that everything would be all right.

I can walk with the confidence of knowing that God will take care of everything. I can lean on God and believe that he will do everything that He promises. I can understand that my pain has a purpose. My pain showed me that my relationship with God was stronger than I thought. I leaned on God more than I thought. Tyree saw this in me.

The walk through the shadow of death brought me closer to God and built my faith and trust in God more. It helped me to rely on God more. How is it possible to walk in the light while walking through the darkest place? My scripture reading brought me to a familiar passage: *"The Lord is my light and my salvation; whom shall I fear."* (Psalm 27:1) It was the light of God that shone in the darkest places to guide my footsteps and kept me on the right path.

It was His strength that helped me to endure the beginning of the death process to its completion. I came out the way God designed for me to come out... with joy and peace. I found joy in following His instructions, leaning toward His will. I trusted the process and it did not take me down. And Tyree is where he desired to be... with

Jesus.

Tyree is no longer in pain. He is no longer suffering from a sickness that the world has no cure for. He is resting until Jesus returns for his church. Do I miss him? Yes, I do. I miss sitting on the porch waving at people who pass by in the cars; eating breakfast on the front porch; or sitting on the porch drinking cold lemonade. Most of all, I miss enjoying each other's company, talking about Jesus, people, our jobs, and the world.

We would cook together, clean the house together, barbeque in the backyard, and landscape together. When he mowed the lawn, I checked on him and made sure he was hydrated because sometimes he would get so caught up in what he was doing that he would forget to drink water. I loved how we watched out for each other.

When I was attending college, he made sure I took breaks to refresh my mind. He made sure I was not disturbed by anything, including phone calls, texts, and him. We agreed when the sewing room door was closed, I was in class. I miss these things, but what I know is that he is in a better place, and I will be in that place when it's my time. In the meantime, God is still the center of my life. I continue to seek first the kingdom of God his righteousness and know that everything will be added unto to me.

Short Prayer

Father God, you did just what you said you would do. I

cannot express with mere words how much I love you, how much I appreciate your love and faithfulness toward me and the world. I pray that your perfect strength continues to operate in me. You are more than enough for me. Thank you, God. Continue to direct my steps and I will continue to listen to you and not myself. In the name of Jesus. Amen.

Scripture

"Trust in the Lord with all thine heart; and lean not unto thine own understanding. In all thy ways acknowledge him, and he shall direct thy paths. (Proverbs 3: 5-6 KJV)

MY GOD IS AWESOME, AND HE'S MORE THAN ENOUGH!

JANET G. MORRIS

ABOUT THE AUTHOR

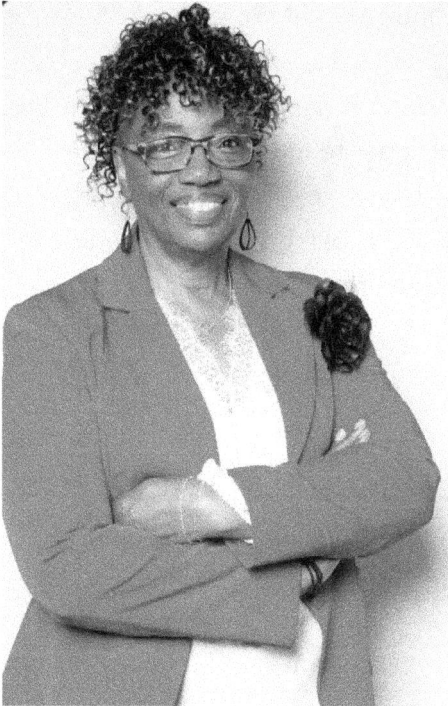

Janet G. Morris is a widow with two sons and eight grandchildren located in the Dallas-Fort Worth Area. She is a retired Senior Workers' Compensation Adjuster who attended Ashford University, where she earned a bachelor's degree in Business with a focus on History and specializing in Human Resources. She obtained her minister license to preach the Gospel in 2003. Janet received a Certificate of Completion from the Simchat Torah Beit Midrash and The International Center for Torah Studies on Ancient Foundations-Volume One. She is Minister-Elder at Radical Remnant Ministries. (Her titles include Evangelist, Superintendent-Sectary of Sunday School, Director of

Vacation Bible School, Youth Director, Usher Board, Women Mission, and Choir. She loves spending time with her family, especially one-on-one time with her grandchildren and currently homeschools one of her three-year-old granddaughters.

Sharing her knowledge and spiritual experiences about God with others shows Janet's passion for others to accept Jesus as their personal savior. It has been stated that, "She is a walking Bible," causing her to delve more into the word of God to share with anyone who chooses to listen. Her hobbies include sewing, cooking, reading, listening to music, drawing, and volunteering. She enjoys seeing action-packed movies on the big screen, sharing Jesus, shopping for her grandchildren, and surprising them with outings and gifts.

Janet has her own constellation by giving her grandchildren names of stars: Singing, Twinkle, Shining, Divine, Amazing, Shooting, Dreaming, and Blessing. She tries to see the good in everyone. Her goal is to strive to live peaceably with everyone and share the love of Christ according to his example. She loves passing out gum and candy to the youth at church. When she worked in the corporate world, she had a candy dish on her desk. If anyone needed a cough drop, she had one to give them. She is always willing to lend a helping hand. She shows the light of Christ everywhere she goes. She endeavors to show the world that there is a better place for all who believe in the Lord Jesus Christ. Janet is kind, sweet, lovable, compassionate, positive, and a very good listener. She's a great motivator, constantly encouraging others and has served in the church for over 50 years.